The Strange Symptoms of Peripheral Neuropathy

Unusual Manifestations of Malfunctioning Nerves as Related by a PN Patient

By: James M. Lowrance © 2013

TABLE OF CONTENTS (Book Length – Approx 4,129 Words):

CHAPTER ONE:
The Burning and Tingling of PN

CHAPTER TWO:
Distinguishing PN from Fibromyalgia

CHAPTER THREE:
Numbness and Proprioception (A Sense of Body Position)

CHAPTER FOUR:
Diabetic "Autonomic Neuropathies" Affecting Bodily Organs and Systems

SUBTITLES:

*The Effects of Temperature Changes on PN
*Negative Nerve Pressure: Impingement
*In My Own Case of PN
*Restless Leg Syndrome
*Where Pain and Other Symptoms Originate between PN and FMS
*The Adrenal Factor
*Slow Healing of Wounds (Usually the Feet)
*Carpal Tunnel Syndrome
*Injuries from Falls
*Functions of the Autonomic Nerves
*Symptoms and Manifestations of Autonomic Neuropathy (AN)
*Case-Examples of Severe AN
*The "Monster Disease" in Patients Who Defy Their PN Treatments

INTRODUCTION:

People who have not personally experienced conditions of "peripheral neuropathy"(PN), will often think that it is simply a condition that causes tingling and burning sensations in the feet, when they hear the term used. This would be correct, however, it is only partially descriptive of PN which can also involve many other things in regard to symptoms.

For some patients, peripheral neuropathy can become seriously disabling and even life-threatening to others. This of course depends on the severity of the disease and how well it has been medically addressed. However, even mild cases of peripheral neuropathy can cause a wide array of physical sensations and problems in people suffering from the varied effects of it.

Over 100 types of PN have been identified, according to medical research organizations.

This demonstrates the fact that each person will experience the physical results of damaged or diseased nerves, differently than do their fellow patients. Some people feel more of the burning sensation while others may feel very strong tingling that literally feels as if a colony of ants are stinging them simultaneously on their feet and/or legs. Some PN patients are affected exclusively within their feet and they may experience not only tingling and burning sensations within them but they may also feel stabbing pains as well. Others may feel pressure type sensations within their feet and/or their hands, as if they are swollen, when they are actually normal size and no fluid retention (edema) is present in them. Yet other PN sufferers may feel a tightening-sensation within their extremities, as if they are wrapped tightly with spandex bandages or they are wearing tight-fitting socks or gloves.

While PN can affect the upper and/or lower extremities, these are certainly not exclusive to the disease.

The trunk of the body can also be involved and all organs inside the body can potentially be involved as well. This is usually the case with nerve damage or neurological diseases that are severe and widespread within the body (systemic) or that involve conditions such as fibromyalgia.

This means that physical sensations may not be the only manifestation of PN but other signs of the disease can include hypo-functioning of bodily organs (the inadequate operation of them) and even a complete failure of them in extreme cases. This would include effects that can occur within the kidneys, the heart and the lungs.

Within the chapters that follow, I will discuss some of the challenges presented to PN patients, resulting from mild, moderate and severe PN symptom-manifestations. I will also relate some of my personal experiences with the disease as I continue through each chapter.

I will not be discussing "causes" for the disease specifically in this particular written work but readers can find more about causes and treatments in my companion book titled: *"Peripheral Neuropathy Causes and Treatments"*. To my surprise, of my approximate 75 published written works, my original peripheral neuropathy book, has been my largest seller since it was published in late 2010. This revealed to me that it addresses a very common and rapidly-growing health problem.

My purpose for this new book/eBook is to help patients with PN conditions know that they are not alone with the sometimes strange and unusual symptoms of their disease, and to help those with friends or loved ones who are sufferers, understand how diverse and sometimes severe symptoms of nerve-related diseases can actually be.

CHAPTER ONE:

The Burning and Tingling of PN

These two symptoms are the most common and for most people with PN, they are usually worse at night and at bedtime before going to sleep. There are not always particular things that cause these sensations to flare but possible triggers can include: being on one's feet for lengthy periods of time, temperature changes or sitting in a chair that places prolonged pressure on the legs (usually between the hips and knees). All of these possible triggers require that the nerves be on high alert, to warn of impending dangers to them or to the tissues they are protecting and supplying with nerve-impulse energy. The person with PN is in essence placing the nerves into higher-use with these type scenarios, or a better term might be to say that more stress is being placed on the affected nerves during these times.

The Effects of Temperature Changes on PN

With significant temperature changes of cold to hot or vise-versa, the nerves are required to adjust quickly but when they have already experienced a degree of damage or they are diseased in general, this can be more difficult for them to accomplish. The sensory nerves are the small-fiber type within the body that conduct feelings and sensations to the brain, to protect the body (i.e. knowing when something is hot enough to burn you or cold enough to cause you frost bite). If they can no longer successfully transmit these feelings, a person may instead simply feel tingling, pin-prick sensations, stabbing pains, waves of chills running up their legs or shock sensations.

Other people with PN, eventually lose the ability with some sensory nerves, to feel temperature or pain sensations at all and they will rather feel a numbness that places them at danger for potential injuries they are unaware of.

This is due to their not knowing if something is occurring to body tissues, such as areas of the feet, that can result in damage to them that may be slow-healing or permanent. Numbness does not always indicate that nerves are severely damaged and can simply manifest in some people with PN, during the early onset of their disease. Strangely, some PN patients feel flares of false cold temperature sensations, as if their feet are freezing rather than burning. The nerve impulses are obviously confused at this point.

Negative Nerve Pressure: Impingement

The issues of remaining on one's feet for lengthy periods of time or of sitting in chairs for prolonged periods that place pressure on the legs, causing PN symptom-flares -- result from crowding the damaged nerves (e.g. constricting, restricting or pinching them). The medical term often used for this is "nerve impingement".

It can also be the result of crowding other nerves that work in cooperation with small fiber nerves, which are the "large fiber nerves". These tie directly into the central nervous system and spinal cord. This is why PN patients often see their symptoms flare with prolonged standing or after sitting in chairs that restrict blood circulation and nerve impulses to the lower legs.

To avoid this in work situations, they usually require restricted periods of standing or sitting, or they will need to take breaks between them if possible. They also require chairs that are well padded up to the knee joints or that allow for propping-up the feet on occasion, which can help to prevent symptoms in the extremities.

Obesity plays a major role as well, in regard to "negative nerve pressure" because having excessive body fat, automatically adds a degree of impingement on the nerves.

In My Own Case of PN

In using my own PN condition as an example; with my being moderately overweight, I can sit in a computer chair that is not well-padded up to the knees and within 20 minutes, I will begin to feel a degree of burning and tingling sensations in my feet. This usually only occurs if a chair lacks proper padding or does not recline to some extent.

I will also feel a sluggishness in the muscles of my legs and feet within a short period of sitting, regardless of the type of chair or seat I'm using. This second type symptom will occur in these muscles for the first couple of minutes after standing to walk even short distances, regardless of how well a chair is padded.

In regard to temperature-changes, my case of PN is not severely affected by changes such as going from warm indoors to very cold outdoors.

My feet however, do seem to be more severely affected by burning and tingling sensations during hot weather and when I am outdoors wearing shoes that are not well-ventilated. I have also noticed that if I use a hot tub indoors during wintertime -- going in with mildly or moderately cool body temperature, into hot water, I can potentially feel very strong tingling sensations in my feet and lower legs. These feel like ant-stings, and because of this I need the temperature of the water adjusted to less-than hot settings. It is during summertime for me, that burning and tingling sensations in my feet become worse at bedtime and during nighttime sleep periods.

Restless Leg Syndrome

For many PN sufferers, Restless Leg Syndrome (RLS), which can be a manifestation of damaged or diseased nerves within the legs or simply from hyperactive nerves, theirs does not correlate with burning and tingling sensations.

This is true in my case as well; my RLS may or may not be accompanied by these other sensations, at any given time when it is flaring. Strangely, my RLS may also flare during the daytime when I am not actively on my feet, and so it is not exclusive to bedtime. I have noticed that these other sensations may or may not be present with my RLS (e.g. burning and tingling) and so the degree of restless leg doesn't correlate in any specific way with other sensory symptoms I may experience. This of course will not be true of other PN patients and some will see all of these symptoms change in severity, simultaneously -- which points to how diverse the disease can be among different patients.

It is possible that the RLS aspect may depend on the root-cause of PN, such as whether or not it is caused by a metabolic disease, by an inflammatory autoimmune disease or by a nutritional deficiency of some type. In some cases, PN may result from a combination of these causes.

CHAPTER TWO:

Distinguishing PN from Fibromyalgia

Fibromyalgia Syndrome (FMS), is a condition in which sufferers of it will experience widespread muscle pain and tender points (areas on the body that experience pain with mild finger-point pressure). Other symptoms are usually present as well, including fatigue, unusual headaches and other sensory changes, such as sensitivity to light in the eyes and intolerance to loud noises coming into the ears.

FMS patients also commonly experience emotional imbalances such as clinical depression and anxiety disorders. According to medical research that has been undertaken in regard to the causes and manifestations of FMS, the syndrome is thought to be the result of amplified pain signals from the nerves and not from them being damaged as occurs with peripheral neuropathy.

With this said, FMS and PN can manifest very similarly, and in some cases they are co-morbid to each other as well (both can occur at the same time). It has been suggested by some MDs who have attended my own medical needs over the past 10 years (since year 2003), that my pain disorder may be a combination of PN and FMS. Chronic Fatigue Syndrome has also been suggested as a possibility in my case (it has 75% crossover similarities to FMS according to reputable medical sources).

An unusual manifestation of my nerve-related symptoms, is sensitivity and tingling that occurs on my scalp -- usually on the top of my head, feeling similar to a sunburn. This last-mentioned symptom I experience, is not typical of PN but is more-so a symptom manifestation reported by FMS patients. This, despite the fact that it would seemingly be a sensory nerve symptom, rather than one of muscle pain.

Again, this shows the diversity of symptoms that can occur between these nerve-related disorders, some of which seem to cross-over at times in some patients. Doctors admit to difficulty in diagnosing some patients who have non-specific or somewhat vague nerve and muscle symptoms and both FMS and CFS are still referred to as "mysterious illnesses" by some medical professionals. Some actually do not recognize these two syndromes as real illnesses, in spite of the fact that they are recognized by the U.S. National Institutes of Health -- Centers for Disease Control (for many years).

Where Pain and Other Symptoms Originate between PN and FMS

Another difference between the two conditions that can help to differentiate between them, is the fact that with FMS, much of the pain being experienced will be within body tissues, namely muscles; while with PN the pain and other nerve-malfunction symptoms are exclusively radiating from damaged nerves.

This is not to say that muscles are not significantly affected by PN, since muscles operate via signals that control them from any affected "motor nerves" but the muscular results of PN is usually found to be a loss of control over them, weakness and muscle loss (atrophy), rather than pain. This would also include trembling and twitches occurring muscularly (fasciculations and tremors), which can be experienced by both FMS and PN patients.

Why small fiber hyper-sensitivity to pain-signals develops in people with FMS, remains a subject of some debate among medical professionals. Some researchers do cite "The Stress Factor" as a possibility, however, meaning that FMS may be a stress-related syndrome. Stress is experienced by all normal human beings and to some extent it is actually normal and healthy, however, severe chronic stress or a traumatic stressful event, can cause FMS and CFS (Chronic Fatigue Syndrome – being a similar condition) to manifest in susceptible individuals.

The Adrenal Factor

While abnormally high levels of stress is not a highly suspected cause of PN, it can still affect patients with nerve damage diseases because it contributes to a diminished ability for the body to maintain an adequate pain threshold (resistance to the effects of pain). Some of this is attributed by medical researchers, to lowered levels of the hormone "cortisol" (also called "cortical"). Some medical studies refer to this condition as "hypocortisolemia". This adrenal stress-hormone, is responsible for helping the body to cope with daily stressors on an ongoing basis. Chronic or traumatic stress however, can place added-demands for adrenal production of cortisol, leading to eventual "low reserves" of the hormone.

This would not be the same as an actual cortisol deficiency, which is found in people with actual adrenal gland diseases (true adrenal deficiency: "Addison's Disease") but it would rather be called an "insufficiency" or low levels that are subclinical.

Some medical sources also refer to mild adrenal insufficiency, as "Adrenal Fatigue" (others do not recognize the condition). With properly-charged adrenal glands being a possible advantage against both FMS and PN, I would suggest that it may be important to maintain good adrenal health. I address more about the connection of Adrenal Fatigue to CFS and FMS, in my book/eBook titled: *"The Best Darn CFS, Fibromyalgia and Adrenal Fatigue Book/eBook"*.

CHAPTER THREE:

Numbness Proprioception (A Sense of Body Position) and Slow Healing

Numbness in cases of PN, of course means that certain body parts have lost the ability to fully feel sensations of temperature-changes and pain.

People with nerve damage diseases, can actually injure their feet for example, or develop ulcers and/or blisters on them, without being aware that they have done so.

Slow Healing of Wounds (Usually the Feet)

I have heard examples of people with numbness from PN, who received cuts on the bottom of their feet while walking on beaches. Because they were unaware of these, their wounds would fester and become infected over time resulting in the need for medical attention.

If they had become aware of their wounds at the time of occurrence, they would likely have been able to avert the need for professional medical care, by simply applying first-aid to their wounds at home.

In the case of my oldest brother, who also has peripheral neuropathy that is "idopathic" like mine (meaning it is not caused by one specific, determined factor), he developed a small blister on one of the smaller toes of his right foot. He was unaware of the need to have the wound attended by a medical doctor and over time the sore became infected and would not begin a healing process. Eventually, infection also entered into the bone of his toe and his doctor had to refer him for toe amputation surgery. He was required to have the toe removed at the bottom-knuckle that adjoins to his foot. This demonstrates the fact that people with numbness from PN, should examine their feet for wounds or blisters that they may be unaware of, to prevent a more serious problem from resulting.

Carpal Tunnel Syndrome

"Carpal Tunnel Syndrome" is a localized median nerve entrapment causing symptoms in the wrist, hand and forearm and can be a type of "mononeuropathy", when it affects only one arm on a person. Some individuals (myself included) experience occasional or frequent difficulty with this type of PN. They will find that they are not gripping objects as firmly as they think (proprioception) and this will cause them to drop things. This is especially true if they are looking-away from their hand position, so that they don't visually see that their grip has loosened on the object they are holding. Some people with carpal tunnel, find it difficult to hold a coffee cup or to control their handwriting so that it appears legible. While I do not experience the actual syndrome, I do have median nerve-weakness in both of my arms. This was revealed on nerve conduction studies as well, that were conducted by my neurologist in the year 2010.

I find that my arm weakness can flare to the point that I find difficulty with handwriting at times but I am grateful that I do not experience pain in my hands as often or as severely as I did before my PN began being treated (mine is "polyneuropathy", affecting both arms and both legs).

Injuries from Falls

The more serious problems that can occur with PN related proprioception, is when it causes patients with nerve disease, to fall when they become unaware of their foot-placement. This can happen while they are climbing flights of stairs and can be due to degrees of numbness and weakness they experience as a result of their PN. In some cases, patients fall while simply walking on carpets or even on level, hard floors which can result in bodily injuries that are severe or even life-threatening (i.e. hip and skull fractures).

It is important for PN patients to know when they are in need of devices that help them to walk more steadfastly, such as the use of canes and/or therapeutic shoes, such as those designed for diabetics.

CHAPTER FOUR:

Diabetic "Autonomic Neuropathies" Affecting Bodily Organs and Systems

Of the three types of nerves that can be affected by PN, the least commonly affected to degrees of true significance (full blown – overt involvement), are the autonomic nerves. This fact however, should not make the following of a doctor's treatment-plan, to control major contributing factors to PN, including diabetes (the "Number One Cause"), any less of a priority. Please read on to understand this warning about the potential for PN patients to develop Autonomic Neuropathies and how severe this disease can potentially become.

Functions of the Autonomic Nerves

While sensory nerves provide normal feelings to the body and motor nerves help with muscle strength and coordination, the autonomic nerves are part of "The Involuntary Nervous System".

This is the part of the system that regulates organs and involuntary responses that occur within the body. This includes heart rate and blood pressure changes needed with correlating changes in physical activity and body posture, in addition to breathing regulation during sleep via the pulmonary system (lungs). It includes the digestive process and body temperature regulation as well, via the amount of fluids retained in the body and released through the sweat glands, salivary ducts and mucous glands. It includes the filtering of impurities from the body as well, with help of the liver and kidneys.

Symptoms and Manifestations of Autonomic Neuropathy (AN)

When cases of PN begin to involve the autonomic nerves, the condition is referred to as "Autonomic Neuropathy" (AN). Some cases of the condition may remain relatively mild during the lifetime of a patient experiencing it, while others may see it progress to moderate and severe levels.

At this point, patients are closely monitored by their treating doctors, in order to detect any indications that organs within the body are beginning to fail. Patients who only see mild manifestations of AN, may only experience things such as increased or decreased sweating, dizziness upon first standing up, urinary or bowel incontinence and impotence in males.

Severe cases of AN however, can lead to conditions such as heart failure, kidney disease (renal failure) and difficulty breathing. When these conditions occur, patients may be referred for pacemaker implantation, kidney dialysis or help with pulmonary function, via oxygen supplementation and/or a ventilator apparatus (breathing machine).

One famous sufferer of diabetic neuropathy, was the beloved musician and singer -- Johnny Cash, who passed away at the age of 71 years (on September 12, 2003), due to respiratory failure caused by AN.

Case-Examples of Severe AN

I will also relate the fact that I have a first-cousin, whose severe, badly-controlled diabetes evolved into severe kidney failure. Because of this, she has been required to receive kidney dialysis on a frequent basis, for approximately two years at the time of this writing. At one point, she was referred for kidney removal, due to one of them becoming so diseased, that it was poisoning her body and the dialysis was no longer helping to the degree it was needed, to filter-out these impurities in her blood. She has since regained some of her health and she remains improved.

I am reminded of an acquaintance I made with a lady at a hospital where I was having a blood draw performed. While in the waiting room, this woman struck up a conversation with me, describing that her AN was near the final stages and that her doctors informed her that her days were limited.

She was in a wheelchair and she informed me that she had just completed a hospital stay, in which they drained large amounts of fluid from her heart, which was in a state of failure (enlargement). Her descriptions of how severe her AN had become as a result of badly-controlled diabetes was disturbing to me. She appeared to be in her 50s and she did not appear to be overweight and yet she told me that she had not been taking care of herself since being diagnosed as a diabetic many years previous.

The "Monster Disease" in Patients Who Defy Their PN Treatments

This kind lady asked if I was checked for diabetes, for which I responded that I certainly had been and that the results were negative for the disease. She then asked if I had family members with the disease for which I replied that yes, I had three extended family members with varied severity of diabetic PN conditions.

She advised me to warn them, with what I had learned from her about what she called "The Monster Disease" and I assured her that I would certainly do so, for those who I knew would listen.

I will say frankly to the readers of this resource, that one of these extended family members I mentioned to this kind lady, refuses to properly control their severe diabetes.

They remain morbidly obese, they do not get the proper types of exercise and they consume things in their diet, that their doctors have placed off-limits to them, including large amounts of refined sugars.

They are literally a time-bomb, that is ready to explode at any time and it saddens me that they refuse to follow their treatment plan, in addition to taking their medications.

It is my hope that this short subject resource, has not only served to inform the readers of it, about some of the strange and unusual symptoms that can occur with PN, but also that it has served as a warning about how severe the disease can become in people who do not follow their doctor's treatment plans.

Sincerely,
Jim Lowrance

Printed in Great Britain
by Amazon